POCKET CLINICAL EXAMINER

Adam Barnett
MA(Cantab) BM BCh
Barts and The London School of Anaesthesia
London, UK

Thomas Bannister
MA(Oxon) BM BCh
Medical Officer, Royal Air Force
UK

T0134033

CRC Press
Taylor & Francis Group
6000 Broken Sound Parkway NW, Suite 300
Boca Raton, FL 33487-2742

Printed in the UK by Severn, Gloucester on responsibly sourced paper
Version Date: 20140407

International Standard Book Number-13: 978-1-4441-7239-3 (Paperback)

Visit the Taylor & Francis Web site at
http://www.taylorandfrancis.com

and the CRC Press Web site at
http://www.crcpress.com

CONTENTS

FOREWORD

For over a decade, Oxford medical students entering the clinical years of the course have been helped through their first fortnight on the wards by senior medical students, who act as tutors, mentors and friends. These trained teachers (colloquially known as 'Med Eds') take responsibility for designing a programme for this crucial introductory period. As well as inducting the students into the culture and practices of the hospital, the tutors introduce the key clinical skills of history and examination. This programme is consistently one of the highest rated parts of the medical course.

A small handbook to support this teaching was an early product of the scheme, and over the years each new cohort of students has improved and refined this resource. I am delighted that Adam Barnett and Tom Bannister, two of our recent graduates and former Med Eds, have taken this process one step further by publishing this textbook, which draws on the accumulated contributions of hundreds of Oxford medical students. It will be a valuable support for medical students anywhere who seek a student-focussed and concise reference source to guide them through acquiring and practising their clinical skills on the wards.

Tim Lancaster
Director of Clinical Studies
Oxford Medical School
Oxford, UK

PREFACE

This book started life as a guide for new Oxford clinical students. Each year it was rewritten by final year medical students, refined, re-imagined, and passed on. We gratefully acknowledge its origins and thank the generations of students on whose shoulders we stand. Without them, we ourselves would not be doctors today!

This little book was so helpful to us and our colleagues during our training that we thought: why not bring it to a wider audience? We want this book to be a loyal companion for the intrepid medical student venturing onto the wards. Whether you're revising for an OSCE, or frantically trying to remember how to do an abdominal examination before a tutorial with a fearsome surgeon, we hope our offering gets you out of all manner of tight spots!

It's not intended to be an exhaustive guide to clinical examination – you can keep that on your shelf at home. Rather, it presents each system examination in a concise, yet comprehensive, 'check sheet' format – and it can easily slip into your pocket. We've tried to highlight common pitfalls and provide useful tips, and have also included sections on history taking, the clerking examination and presenting your findings.

We'd like to thank all of the unnamed students who have contributed to this book. We are also deeply indebted to Drs Charlotte Bendon, Nina Dutta, Lydia Hanna, Nadeem Hasan, Andrew Jones and Rebecca Mills for contributing individual chapters. We'd also like to thank the kind folk at Hodder/Taylor & Francis for their forbearance and wisdom.

Above all, though, we'd like to thank you, the reader. We hope that you find this book useful and even (whisper it) fun! If you've got any ideas as to how we can improve it, please do get in touch.

We should emphasise that any errors in this book are entirely our own.

CONTRIBUTORS

Charlotte Lucy Bendon BA BM BCh MRCS
Core Surgical Trainee
Oxford Deanery, UK

Nina Dutta BM BCh MA DRCOG MRCP
General Practice Specialist Trainee
Riverside Scheme
London, UK

Lydia Hanna MBBS BSc(Anat) MRCS
Core Surgical Trainee
Kent, Surrey, Sussex Deanery, UK

Nadeem Hasan BM BCh MA MSc DRCOG DFPH
Specialty Registrar in Public Health
London Deanery, UK

Andrew Richard Jones MBBS BSc MRCS
Core Surgical Trainee
Wales Deanery, UK

Rebecca Mills BM BCh MA MRCS
Core Surgical Trainee
London Deanery, UK

ABOUT THE AUTHORS

Adam Barnett is an ACCS (Anaesthetics) CT1 trainee at Barts and The London School of Anaesthesia. He recently took a year out of training, working as a NICU registrar in Australia, and in Cambodia as part of NHS South's Improving Global Health through Leadership Development programme. He studied medicine at Cambridge and Oxford, and did his foundation years in the Oxford deanery. During 2011–2012 he was lecturer in medicine at Queen's College, Oxford.

Tom Bannister is currently a GP trainee with the Royal Air Force. He read medicine at Oxford, where he spent almost as much time teaching as he did learning. He was the Jesus College tutor in Pathology from 2008 to 2010, taught a course in inter-professional communication skills and founded an OSCE training weekend for 4th year students.

ABBREVIATIONS

ACL	anterior cruciate ligament
ACS	acute coronary syndrome
ADL	activities of daily living
AP	anteroposterior
AV	atrioventricular
β-hCG	beta-human chorionic gonadotrophin
BMI	body mass index
BS	bowel sounds
CABG	coronary artery bypass graft
CO	carbon monoxide
CO_2	carbon dioxide
COPD	chronic obstructive pulmonary disease
CRP	C-reactive protein
CRT	capillary refill time
CVS	cardiovascular system
DHx	drug history
DKA	diabetic ketoacidosis
DVT	deep vein thrombosis
ECG	electrocardiogram
FHx	family history
FNA	fine-needle aspiration
GCS	Glasgow Coma Scale
GI	gastrointestinal
GP	general practitioner
GTN	glyceryl trinitrate
GU	genitourinary
HPC	history of presenting complaint
HRT	hormone replacement therapy
IPJ	interphalangeal joint
IV	intravenous
IVDU	intravenous drug use
JVP	jugular venous pressure

LCL	lateral cruciate ligament
LMN	lower motor neuron
MCL	medial cruciate ligament
MCP	metacarpophalangeal
MRC	Medical Research Council
NBM	nil by mouth
NG	nasogastric
NHS	National Health Service
NKDA	no known drug allergies
O_2	oxygen
OA	osteoarthritis
OSCE	objective structured clinical examination
PC	presenting complaint
PCA	patient-controlled analgesia
PCL	posterior cruciate ligament
PMHx	past medical history
SE	systems enquiry
SHx	social history
SVC	superior vena cava
TED	thromboembolic deterrent
TPN	total parenteral nutrition
U&E	urea and electrolytes
UMN	upper motor neuron
UTI	urinary tract infection

Chapter 1

Taking a History

Introduction and consent	For example: 'Hello, Mr/Mrs/Ms . . .; my name is . . .. I am a (medical student/doctor/etc.). May I ask you some questions?'
Confirm patient details	• Name • Gender • Age • Date of birth (Note that this also acts as a quick check of the patient's cognitive state.)
Presenting complaint (PC)	'Why have you come into hospital?' You should record this in the patient's own words (e.g. 'shortness of breath' rather than 'dyspnoea').

NB – A patient may have more than one presenting complaint. If you feel that they can be grouped together (e.g. diarrhoea and vomiting) then do so. If not, record them separately, number them and take a separate history of the presenting complaint for each.

| History of presenting complaint (HPC) | <ul><li>Start by letting the patient tell you his or her story in an 'open-ended' manner. *'When were you last well?'* and *'What has happened since then?'* are useful questions.</li><li>Then seek clarification/additional information as required, e.g. for diarrhoea:<ul><li>for how long?</li><li>how many episodes per day?</li><li>is there any blood in it?</li><li>was there a fever?</li><li>has the patient travelled recently?, etc.</li></ul></li><li>With practice you will learn what the relevant, specific questions are for each presentation.</li></ul>A useful general framework is **'SIC CARERS'**:<ul><li>**S**tart: when did it start?</li><li>**I**nterim: what has happened since then?</li><li>**C**urrently: what is the situation like now?</li></ul> |

HPC	• **C**haracter: what is the precise nature
(continued)	of the complaint, e.g. for vomiting:
	○ what does it look like?
	○ any blood, etc.
	• **A**ssociated symptoms.
	• **R**elievers: does anything make it
	better?
	• **E**xacerbants: does anything make it
	worse?
	• **R**isk factors: for example, for
	chest pain ask about cardiac risk
	factors; any hypertension/diabetes/
	hypercholesterolaemia/smoking/
	personal or family history of heart
	disease, etc.?
	• **S**ystem enquiry: ask about the
	relevant organ system (e.g.
	GI for vomiting; see 'Systems enquiry'
	section).

'SOCRATES' is frequently used for taking an HPC of a pain:

- **S**ite: where is the pain?
- **O**nset: sudden or gradual?
- **C**haracter: *'Can you describe the pain?'* (tight band/sharp/burning dull ache, etc.)
- **R**adiation: does the pain move elsewhere?
- **A**ssociated symptoms: shortness of breath, nausea, vomiting, fever, etc.

HPC *(continued)*	• **Timing:** how long does it last; does it come and go, or is it constant? • **Exacerbants/relievers:** does anything make it better or worse? • **Severity:** *'Can you rate your pain out of ten, where one is barely there, and ten is the worst pain imaginable? Does it prevent you from doing anything?'*
Past medical history (PMHx)	This information relates to past illnesses, operations, admissions to hospital, and the like. • *'Do you have any other medical problems'* and *'Do you see your GP regularly for any reason?'* are useful questions. • Be persistent; it is often surprising what patients will forget. Ask specifically about **'MJ THREADS PD'** (**m**yocardial infarction, **j**aundice, **t**uberculosis, **h**ypertension, **r**heumatic fever, **e**pilepsy, **a**sthma, **d**iabetes, **s**troke, **p**ulmonary embolus and **d**eep vein thrombosis).
Drug history (DHx)	Drug allergies and intolerances *'What happens when you take the drug?'* If no drug allergies, record 'NKDA'.

BEWARE – Patients sometimes believe that they have an allergy when they do not; vomiting is not an allergic reaction.

DHx
(continued)
	Current medications
	Includes prescriptions (including the oral contraceptive pill), over-the-counter medicines and herbal supplements (especially St John's wort).
	• For each medication, record:
	   ○ drug.
	   ○ dose and route.
	   ○ indication.
	   ○ date started.
	• Questions to ask include:
	   ○ *'Do you actually take all of the regular medications prescribed for you?'*
	   ○ *'Have you recently changed, started or stopped any medications?'*
	   ○ *'Do you take any recreational drugs?'*

Family history (FHx)	*'Are there any illnesses that run in the family?'* Ask specifically about heart attacks, diabetes and malignancy. If there is an extensive family history, you might want to draw a family tree.

Social history (SHx)	Include current/former occupations.

Living situation and care needs

'What type of house do you live in (e.g. does it have stairs)?'

'Who do you live with?' is a useful question in order to find out if there is care available for the patient, if required.

- Is the patient themselves a carer?
- ADL: are they independent with washing, dressing, etc.? Do they have a package of care?
- Mobility: do they require walking aids/a wheelchair?

Smoking

'Do you smoke?' and (if not) *'Have you ever smoked?'*

'How many years did you smoke in total?' is a useful question.

Quote smoking history in 'pack-years' (20 cigarettes per day for 1 year = 1 'pack-year').

Alcohol

If there is a significant alcohol history, ask if they have ever tried stopping completely, if they have had seizures related to alcohol, or if they have been admitted to the hospital with complications of their alcoholism.

SHx *(continued)*	Also potentially relevant: hobbies, pets, recent travel, etc.
Systems enquiry (SE)	General Fever, unintentional weight loss (how much, over what time period), night sweats, change of appetite, fatigue/lethargy/malaise. Cardiovascular system (CVS) Chest pain, palpitations, ankle swelling, orthopnoea, paroxysmal nocturnal dyspnoea. Respiratory Hoarseness, cough, shortness of breath, haemoptysis, wheeze. Gastrointestinal Dysphagia, reflux, nausea, vomiting, change in bowel habit, blood or mucus in stool. Genitourinary (GU) Frequency, urgency, dysuria, nocturia, haematuria. • Men: hesitancy, terminal dribbling, poor stream, impotence. • Women: discharge, itch, timing and character of menses.

SE (continued)	Neurological 'Fits/faints/funny turns', falls, numbness, tingling, weakness, unusual headaches, visual disturbances. Musculoskeletal Joint or muscle aches, joint swelling or stiffness, rashes.
Closure	Thank the patient and make sure that the patient is comfortable.

TO FINISH

At the end of each stage of the history, a useful tool is to summarise what has been elicited thus far. That way, the patient can correct any misunderstandings, and you can ask if there is anything you have missed. It also shows that you have been listening to what the patient has been saying.

Chapter 2

Examination of the Cardiovascular System

TO START	
WIPE:	
Wash your hands.	
Introduce yourself to the patient.	
Permission: ask to examine the patient.	
Position: start with the patient sitting at 45°.	
Pain: check that the patient has no pain.	
Exposure: top off (women can keep their bra on, but be careful not to miss an underlying scar).	
End of the bed	Surroundings
	• Monitoring: ECG, observations.
	• Treatments: O_2, infusions, vascular access, GTN spray, TED stockings, insulin pen, etc.
	Patient
	Sick or well?

End of the bed *(continued)*	Alert or drowsy? Obese? Short of breath? Pale? Malar flush? Sternotomy scar? Pacemaker?

Cardiac risk factors

- Smoking.
- Diabetes.
- Hypertension.
- Hypercholesterolaemia.
- Personal history of cardiovascular disease.
- Strong family history of cardiovascular disease.
- Increasing age.
- Male sex.

Hands	Are the hands warm and well-perfused?
	Nails • Clubbing. • Splinter haemorrhages: trauma or bacterial endocarditis (<3 is normal). • CRT test at the level of the heart (<2 seconds is normal). Hands • Osler's nodes, Janeway lesions: bacterial endocarditis. • Pale palmar creases: anaemia. • Tendon xanthomata: familial hypercholesterolaemia.

Arms	Look for: track marks (IVDU); tattoos (endocarditis risk); and scars (e.g. radial artery harvest for CABG).
	Radial pulse
	• Rate: count for 15 s then multiply by 4.
	• Rhythm: regular, regularly irregular, or irregularly irregular (atrial fibrillation).
	• Collapsing pulse: aortic regurgitation.
	• Radioradial difference.
	• Radiofemoral delay.
	Measure the blood pressure (ideally in both arms).
Face	Eyes
	• Corneal arcus: normal in the elderly, hyperlipidaemia in young people.
	• Pale conjunctiva: anaemia.
	• Conjunctival petechial haemorrhages: bacterial endocarditis.
	• Xanthelasma: hyperlipidaemia.
	Mouth
	• Mucous membranes: hydration status.
	• Under the tongue: central cyanosis.
	• Poor dentition: bacterial endocarditis risk.
Neck	Carotid pulse
	• Volume: normal, high volume, low volume.

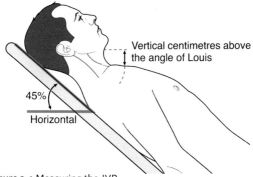

Vertical centimetres above the angle of Louis

45%

Horizontal

Figure 2.1 Measuring the JVP.

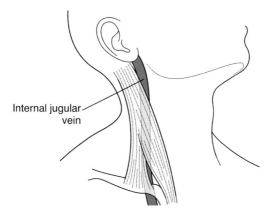

Internal jugular vein

Figure 2.2 The course of the internal jugular vein in relation to the sternocleidomastoid and the clavicle.

Neck *(continued)*	• Character: normal, collapsing, slow rising.
	Jugular venous pressure (JVP)
	Measure with the patient sitting at 45°. Find the vertical distance between the angle of Louis (manubriosternal angle) and the top of the JVP (Figs 2.1, 2.2). It is normally <3 cm.
Precordium	Inspection
	• Scars: sternotomy (likely CABG or valve replacement), posterolateral thoracotomy (e.g. mitral valve surgery), pacemaker (usually below left clavicle).
	• Visible apex beat.
	Palpation
	• Apex: normally in the left fifth intercostal space, midclavicular line (often just below the nipple).
	• Palpable/impalpable?
	• Character: normal, sustained (increased afterload), double impulse (palpable third or fourth heart sound).
	• Position: normal, displaced (cardiomegaly).
	• Parasternal heave: press firmly to feel for ventricular hypertrophy.

Precordium *(continued)*	• Thrills: press lightly over the base of the heart to detect palpable murmurs.
	Auscultation (Fig. 2.3) Listen whilst feeling the carotid pulse. At each area, try to identify:
	• First heart sound: AV valves closing.
	• Second heart sound: aortic/ pulmonary valves closing.
	• Third heart sound: rapid ventricular filling.
	• Fourth heart sound: atrial contraction against a non-compliant ventricle.
	• Additional sounds: prosthetic valves.
	• Murmurs: listen in systole, listen in diastole.

Auscultation areas

Referring to the cardiac auscultation areas anatomically (lower left sternal edge) avoids confusing tautology; for instance, when describing the murmur of aortic regurgitation as a diastolic murmur heard best in the 'tricuspid' area (lower left sternal edge).

	Diaphragm of stethoscope (high-pitched sounds)
	• Apex ('mitral' area).
	• Lower left sternal edge ('tricuspid' area).
	• Upper left sternal edge ('pulmonary' area).
	• Upper right sternal edge ('aortic' area).

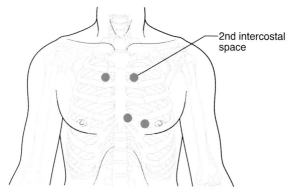

2nd intercostal space

Figure 2.3 Points for auscultation of heart sounds: upper right sternal edge, upper left sternal edge, lower left sternal edge, apex.

Precordium (continued)	If you hear a murmur: track radiation into axilla/carotids.
	Bell of stethoscope (low-pitched sounds: press gently)
	• Carotid bruits: patient should hold their breath and so should you.
	• Apex.
	Dynamic manoeuvres: for diastolic murmurs
	• The bell is in place over the apex, the patient rolls into the left lateral position with the left hand behind the head. Breath is held in expiration (mitral stenosis).

Precordium *(continued)*	• The patient sits forwards; listen at the lower left sternal edge with the diaphragm. Breath is held in expiration (aortic regurgitation). • With the patient still sitting forwards, listen at lung bases: ○ crepitations (overload), reduced air entry (pleural effusion). Palpate for sacral oedema: put the bed flat and lie the patient down.
Abdomen	• Shifting dullness: ascites. • Palpate the liver: hepatomegaly in right heart failure, pulsatile enlarged liver in tricuspid regurgitation.
Legs	• Inspect for longitudinal scars (e.g. long saphenous vein for bypass grafting). • Palpate for pitting oedema. • Glance at the feet (e.g. clubbing, signs of embolism).
Closure	• Thank the patient. • Make sure the patient is comfortable and clothed. • Wash your hands.

TO FINISH

If relevant to findings so far:

Examinations

Complete examination of peripheral vascular system.

Take blood pressure in both arms (aortic dissection or coarctation).

Take lying and standing blood pressures (normal <20 mmHg systolic and <10 mmHg diastolic difference).

Fundoscopy: hypertensive changes, diabetic changes, Roth spots (bacterial endocarditis).

Bedside tests

ECG.

O_2 saturation.

Urine dipstick (blood and protein: hypertension, bacterial endocarditis, etc.).

Investigations

Chest X-ray (e.g. signs of congestive heart failure).

Blood (choice of tests dependent on differential diagnosis).

Chapter 3

Examination of the Respiratory System

TO START	
WIPE:	
Wash your hands.	
Introduce yourself to the patient.	
Permission: ask to examine the patient.	
Position: start with the patient sitting at 45°.	
Pain: check that the patient has no pain.	
Exposure: top removed.	
End of the bed	Surroundings
	• Treatments: O_2 (note method and rate of delivery; see Table 3.1, p.24), inhalers, nebulisers, etc.
	• Paraphernalia: sputum pots, cigarettes, etc.
	Patient
	Sick or well?
	Alert and orientated? Confused?
	Drowsy?

End of the bed *(continued)*	Obvious shortness of breath? Cyanosed (blue)? Coughing? Obvious stridor/wheeze? Cachectic?
Hands ('5 Cs')	**C**lubbing. **C**yanosis (peripheral). **C**igarette tar stains. '**C**ancer': apical lung tumour can cause wasting of the small muscles of the hand (look for dorsal guttering, especially of first dorsal interosseous). **C**O_2 retention flap: ask the patient to cock a wrist back and look for flap. You can also feel the radial pulse at the same time.
Arms	Radial pulse (with CO_2 retention flap; see 'Hands').
Face	• Colour: cyanosis (lips, peripheral cyanosis; under tongue, central cyanosis); plethora (smokers, SVC obstruction [e.g. compression by lung tumour]); pallor; bright red (CO poisoning). • Conjunctival pallor: anaemia. • Horner's syndrome (unilateral ptosis, miosis and anhidrosis); may be from an apical lung tumour.

Neck	• JVP; see Chapter 2, Examination of the Cardiovascular System). • Tracheal deviation. • Cervical and supraclavicular lymphadenopathy.
Chest	Inspection • Scars: thoracotomy (pneumonectomy, lobectomy, etc.); chest drains. • Radiotherapy stigmata: tattoos, skin changes. • Shape: pectus excavatum/carinatum, barrel chest, kyphoscoliosis. • Expansion: symmetry, depth. Palpation • Expansion: anteroposterior ('pump handle') and lateral ('bucket handle'). • Apex beat. • Right ventricular heave. Percussion • Midclavicular line: upper, middle and lower lung fields. • Midaxillary line: lung bases. • Compare right with left. Auscultation • Ask the patient to breathe in and out normally through the mouth. • Listen for a full respiratory cycle at each point.

Chest *(continued)*	• Auscultate at the same points as for percussion.
	• Compare right with left (Fig. 3.1).
	• Breath sounds:
	  ○ air entry: good, reduced or absent.
	  ○ quality: vesicular (normal)/ bronchial.
	• Added sounds:
	  ○ crackles (also known as crepitations), wheeze, pleural rub (like 'shoes in the snow').
	  (See Table 3.2, p.25.)
	• Vocal resonance:
	  'Say 'ninety-nine' every time I place my stethoscope on your chest.'
	  ○ same areas as for percussion/ auscultation.

Back	Repeat percussion and auscultation as previously.
NB – The greater part of the lung bases are at the back.	
	Also palpate for sacral oedema.
Legs	Leg oedema • Bilateral: heart failure (including cor pulmonale). • Unilateral: consider DVT (or lymphoedema if non-pitting).

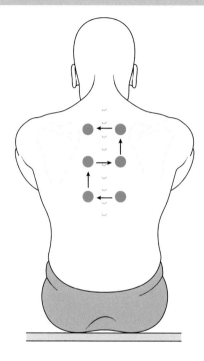

Figure 3.1 AP view of the lungs. Auscultation points on the back. Listen between the thick paraspinal muscles and the scapula. Work from one side to the other, then up, and then across again. This is the easiest way to detect differences between sides and differences within the same lung, such as the fluid level of a pleural effusion.

Closure	• Thank the patient.
	• Make sure the patient is comfortable and clothed.
	• Wash your hands.

TO FINISH

SPOT X:

Sputum sample.

Peak expiratory flow rate measurement.

Oxygen saturations.

Temperature.

X-ray (chest).

NB – This is not a 'one-size-fits-all' list. Further investigations should always be guided by the clinical picture thus far.

TABLE 3.1 Oxygen delivery methods

Method of delivery	Flow rate	Estimated O$_2$ (%)
Nasal cannulae	1–6 L/min (uncomfortable above 4 L/min)	24–40
Hudson mask	10–12 L/min	40–60
Mask with reservoir bag	Up to 15 L/min	80
Mask with Venturi connector (colours and flow rates may vary with manufacturer)	Blue (2 L/min) White (4 L/min) Yellow (8 L/min) Red (10 L/min) Green (15 L/min)	24 28 35 40 60

TABLE 3.2 Interpreting clinical findings

	Expansion	Percussion	Breath sounds	Vocal resonance	Tracheal deviation
Normal	Equal	Normal	Vesicular	Muffled	Central
Consolidation	Reduced	Dull	Bronchial	Increased	Central
Pleural effusion	Reduced	'Stony dull'	Reduced/absent	Reduced/absent	Central/away from affected side
Pneumothorax	Reduced	Hyper-resonant	Reduced/absent	Reduced/absent	Central (simple)/away from affected side (tension)
Collapse	Reduced	Dull	Reduced	Reduced	Towards affected side
Pneumonectomy	Reduced	Dull	Reduced	Increased	Towards affected side
Fibrosis	Reduced	Dull	Reduced	Muffled	Central

Chapter 4

Examination of the Abdominal System

TO START
WIPE:

Wash your hands.

Introduce yourself to the patient.

Permission: ask to examine the patient.

Position: start with the patient sitting at 45°.

Pain: check that the patient has no pain and if the patient would be comfortable to lie completely flat later in the examination.

Exposure: top removed (women can keep their bra on); trouser fly undone and underwear lowered to expose inguinal regions. (Traditionally, exposure is 'nipple to knee,' although this is rarely done in reality.)

End of the bed	Surroundings
	• Monitoring: observations.
	• Paraphernalia: NBM sign, food and drink, vomit bowl.

End of the bed *(continued)*	• Treatments: O_2, infusions, TPN, NG tubes, surgical drains, catheter, TED stockings.
	Patient Sick or well? Alert or drowsy? Cachectic or obese? Comfortable at rest? Writhing (colicky pain)? Very still (peritonism)? Colour: jaundiced (hepatobiliary disease), pale (anaemia), pigmented (haemochromatosis or Addison's disease)?
Hands	Are the hands warm and well-perfused?
	Nails • Clubbing: cirrhosis, inflammatory bowel disease, malabsorption. • Koilonychia: spoon-shaped nails (iron deficiency). • Leuconychia: pale nails (hypoalbuminaemia).
	Hands • Palmar erythema: portal hypertension, chronic liver disease. • Pale palmar creases: anaemia. • Dupuytren's contracture: alcoholic liver disease (many other causes, including idiopathic).

Hands *(continued)*	• Asterixis ('liver flap'): hold arms outstretched with wrists extended for 15 s; observe for a coarse flap rather than fine tremor.

Arms	• Radial pulse: tachycardic?
	• Measure blood pressure.
	• Look for:
	  ○ bruises: impaired clotting factor production in liver disease.
	  ○ excoriations (scratch marks): pruritis secondary to hyperbilirubinaemia.
	  ○ wasting: malignancy?
	• Risk factors for hepatitis: needle track marks, tattoos.

Face	Eyes • Pale conjunctiva: anaemia. • Scleral icterus: yellow tinge to sclera (jaundice). • Kayser–Fleischer rings: copper deposition in Descemet's membrane (at corneal periphery) seen in Wilson's disease. Mouth • Angular stomatitis: B_{12}, folate or iron deficiency. • Ulcers: Crohn's disease or ulcerative colitis.

Face *(continued)*	• Tongue: pale and smooth (iron deficiency), red and beefy (B_{12} and folate deficiency). • Gums and dentition: nutritional status. • Breath: alcohol, DKA ('pear drops'), foetor hepaticus (liver failure).
Neck	• JVP. • Lymphadenopathy: particularly Virchow's node in the left supraclavicular fossa; a palpable node here is Troisier's sign, suggestive of intra-abdominal malignancy (e.g. gastric cancer).
Chest	• Gynaecomastia: breast tissue in males (excess oestrogen in liver disease or as a drug side-effect, such as from spironolactone used for ascites). • Spider naevi: telangiectatic lesions that fill from a central vessel; more than five in the distribution of the superior vena cava is pathological (liver disease).
Back	• Ask the patient to sit forwards: look for scars (e.g. nephrectomy). • Put the bed flat and lie the patient down.

Abdomen	Inspection
	• Scars, wounds, stoma bags, sinuses, striae (stretch marks), bruises, caput medusae (portal hypertension), distension, asymmetry, obvious masses.
	• Ask the patient to take a deep breath in (peritonism).
	• Ask the patient to lift his or her head off the bed whilst you observe for incisional hernias, parastomal hernias or divarication of the rectus abdominis.
	• If the patient has a stoma, comment on position, bag contents, spout and any local irritation or sinus tracts.
	Palpation
	• Ask about pain.
	• Palpate at the level of the patient (i.e. kneel down or raise the bed): start furthest from area of pain, palpating first superficially, then deeply; move systematically through the nine zones (Fig. 4.1), watching the patient's face for pain as you palpate. Define any masses or organomegaly.
	• Tenderness: generalised or localised (define area)?
	• Masses: examine as you would a lump (site, size, shape, etc.).

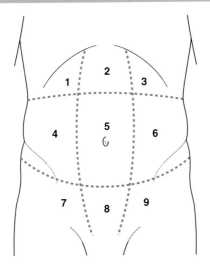

Figure 4.1 The nine sectors of the abdomen.
1: right hypochondrium; 2: epigastrium; 3: left
hypochondrium; 4: right flank; 5: periumbilical region;
6: left flank; 7: right iliac fossa; 8: suprapubic region;
9: left iliac fossa.

Abdomen *(continued)*	• Guarding: voluntary (distractible) or involuntary? • Special signs (if appropriate): Rebound tenderness, Murphy's sign (cholecystitis), Rovsing's sign and McBurney's point tenderness (appendicitis).

| Abdomen *(continued)* | • Organomegaly: liver (palpate from right iliac fossa); spleen (palpate from right iliac fossa; it enlarges diagonally across the abdomen); kidneys (ballot); abdominal aortic aneurysm (palpate deeply in the epigastric region for pulsatile and expansile mass, diameter >3 cm).
• Inguinal hernias: place the fingertips of each hand over the inguinal rings and ask the patient to give a strong cough; note a cough impulse or frank herniation. If a hernia is present, is it reducible (ask the patient to do so initially)? In a male patient with a hernia, examine for scrotal extension of the mass.

Percussion
• Liver, spleen, bladder.
• Shifting dullness (ascites): only perform if the abdomen is distended. (See Table 4.1, p.35.)

Auscultation
• Aortic and renal artery bruits.
• BS: normal, tinkling, absent (normal, obstruction, or ileus, respectively):
   ○ listen for 3 min before concluding BS are absent. |

Closure	• Thank the patient.
	• Make sure the patient is comfortable and clothed.
	• Wash your hands.

TO FINISH

If relevant to findings so far:

Examinations

Formally examine hernial orifices (including femoral) and the external genitalia.

Perform a digital rectal examination.

Examine legs for bruising, oedema and erythema nodosum (associated with inflammatory bowel disease).

Bedside tests

Basic observations.

Urine dip: blood, nitrites and leukocytes in UTI; ketones in DKA; β-hCG in women of child-bearing age (risk of ectopic pregnancy).

Investigations

Abdominal X-ray.

Arterial blood gas: DKA, pancreatitis (modified Glasgow score), ischaemic bowel.

TABLE 4.1 Causes of abdominal distension

Fluid

Fat

Flatus

Faeces

Foetus

Chapter 5

Examination of the Cranial Nerves

You have **24** cranial nerves; remember to test both left and right. The key to a successful cranial nerve examination is to have a slick system and to give clear instructions to the patient. Practice how you will phrase your instructions; it will become apparent in an examination if you have not tested your instructions on real patients.

TO START

WIPE:

Wash your hands.

Introduce yourself to the patient.

Permission: ask *'Please, may I examine the nerves in your face and neck?'*

Position: the patient is seated facing you.

Pain: check that the patient has no pain.

Exposure: whole face and neck.

End of the bed	Surroundings
	Wheelchair, glasses, soft diet or food thickener, NBM sign.
	Patient
	Facial asymmetry (facial nerve palsy or stroke), drooling from one side of the mouth, ptosis.
I: Olfactory	*'Have you noticed a change in your sense of smell or taste recently?'*
	If yes, enquire about a recent cold and check that the nostrils are not physically blocked.
	'I would like to formally assess the sense of smell.' This is rarely done, but you should know how to do so using distinctive aromas, such as coffee or orange peel. Formal kits for testing smell do exist. Remember to test each nostril separately.
II: Optic	Acuity
	'Do you normally use glasses or contact lenses for reading?'
	• Allow the patient to use his or her normal visual aid; you are testing the optic nerve, not the extent of their refractive error.
	• Test each eye in turn; ask the patient to cover the other eye.

| II: Optic *(continued)* | • Ideally, use a Snellen chart at 2.5 m; alternatively, crudely assess vision using a newspaper or your name badge.
• If vision is very poor, try finger counting, detecting hand movements or detecting light.

Fields
• Position yourself opposite the patient approximately 1 m away so you are at the same eye level.
• Hold your finger out equidistant between you and the patient.

'Cover one eye. Look at my nose but tell me when you are aware of my finger moving.'
• Test each visual quadrant in comparison to your own. Start with your finger stationary at the outer edge of each quadrant; offer small movements of the fingertip initially.
• Test macular (central) vision, ideally with a red hat pin.

Reflexes
• Inspect for resting pupil size and symmetry.
• Light reactivity (tests nerves II [afferent] and III [efferent]); note direct and consensual reflexes. |

II: Optic *(continued)*	• Accommodation: pupils should constrict as the patient switches focus from far to near.
	Opthalmoscopy In an OSCE it is normally sufficient simply to offer to do this. However, you should be prepared actually to perform fundoscopy if required. Identify blood vessels and trace them back towards the optic disc. Check for papilloedema and the retinal appearances of diabetes and hypertension.
III, IV, VI: Oculomotor, Trochlear, Abducens	Examine for ptosis, nystagmus and strabismus (squints). *'Do you suffer from double vision?'* Eye movements *'Keep your head still and follow my finger with your eyes.'* • Ensure you pause at the edges of comfortable gaze to inspect for nystagmus. • Ask if the patient gets double vision at any point.
V: Trigeminal	Facial sensation (Fig. 5.1) *'Please shut your eyes. I'm going to gently touch your face on both sides with my fingers. Tell me when you feel me touching you. Does it feel the same on both sides?'*

V: Trigeminal *(continued)*	Stay close to the midline to avoid the C2 dermatome. Motor function *'Please clench your teeth.'* Feel the masseter and temporalis on both sides and assess for symmetry or wasting. *'Now open your jaw. Don't allow me to close it.'* Tests power in the pterygoids. • Offer to perform a jaw jerk: upper motor neuron sign if brisk. • Offer to test the corneal reflex; tests V (afferent) and VII (efferent).

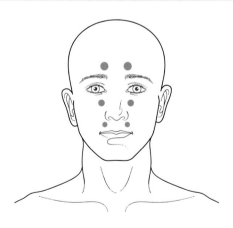

Figure 5.1 Areas for testing the sensory branches of the trigeminal nerve (V).

VII: Facial	Observe closely for asymmetry; it can be subtle: *'Raise your eyebrows.'* *'Close your eyes as tightly as you can.'* *'Blow out your cheeks.'* *'Show me your teeth.'* Note that there is bilateral preganglionic (upper) motor neuron innervation of the forehead. In a lower motor neuron lesion, the muscles of the forehead will be paralysed (such as in Bell's palsy); however, an upper motor neuron lesion (such as a stroke) will spare the forehead.
VIII: Vestibulo-cochlear	*'Can you repeat this number please?'* Whisper a two-digit number in one ear whilst covering, or making a distracting noise in, the other ear. If there is evidence of hearing loss, offer Weber's (256-Hz tuning fork) and Rinne's (512-Hz tuning fork) tests to determine whether the loss is sensorineural or conductive.

Weber's and Rinne's tests

- Sensorineural hearing loss: Weber's test lateralises to the unaffected side. Rinne's test is positive (air conduction is louder than bone conduction, this is normal).

- Conductive hearing loss: Weber's test lateralises to the affected side. Rinne's test is negative (bone conduction is louder than air conduction, this is abnormal)

IX, X, XII: Glossopharyngeal, Vagus, Hypoglossal	*'Open your mouth and say 'Aah'.'* • Illuminate with a pen torch and look for palatal symmetry and uvular deviation (away from the affected side). • Offer to test the gag reflexes (remember both left and right). • Look for wasting or fasciculation of the tongue. *'Stick out your tongue.'* Look for deviation (towards the affected side).
XI: Accessory	*'Shrug your shoulders.'* Check for symmetry; assess trapezius power. *'Turn your head to the right; now, turn back against my hand.'* The sternocleidomastoid turns the head back to the midline; therefore, the patient must turn his or her head first and try to bring it back to a neutral position against resistance. Palpate the contralateral sternocleidomastoid and assess its power. Test the other side as well.
Closure	• Thank the patient. • Make sure the patient is comfortable and clothed. • Wash your hands.

TO FINISH

If relevant to findings so far:
　　Full neurological examination of the limbs.

Chapter 6

Examination of the Neurological System of the Limbs

Always remember: the 'peripheral' neurological examination tests both the peripheral and central nervous systems. The key aim is to identify the anatomical site of the lesion: central versus peripheral. The pattern of signs is usually more important than any one particular sign ('glove-and-stocking' neuropathy, upper motor neuropathy, etc.).

Mnemonic

NB – To Postpone Reflexes Constitutes Stupidity:

    Tone
    Power
    Reflexes
    Coordination
    Sensation

UPPER LIMB EXAMINATION

TO START

WIPE:
Wash your hands.
Introduce yourself to the patient.
Permission: ask to examine the patient.
Position: start with the patient sitting.
Pain: check that the patient has no pain.
Exposure: both upper limbs from shoulders to fingers.

End of the bed	Surroundings
	• Monitoring: cardiac (autonomic problems).
	• Treatments: O_2, infusions (e.g. intravenous immunoglobulin), ventilation.
	• Paraphernalia: wheelchair, mobility aids.
	Patient
	• Asymmetry, deformity or abnormal posture.
	• Resting tremor.
	• Wasting: especially first dorsal interosseous, deltoid, supra- and infraspinatus.
	• Fasciculation: especially anterior deltoid margin and first dorsal interosseous.

Movement	Primary muscle[a]	Root	Nerve
Shoulder abduction	Deltoid	C5	Axillary
Elbow flexion	Biceps	C5, C6	Musculocutaneous
Elbow extension	Triceps	C7	Radial
Wrist flexion	Flexor carpi radialis and ulnaris	C8	Median and ulnar
Wrist extension	Extensor carpi radialis and ulnaris	C7	Radial and posterior interosseous
Finger abduction	Dorsal interossei and abductor digiti minimi	T1	Ulnar
Thumb abduction	Abductor pollicis brevis	C8	Median

[a] Other muscles may also contribute.

Tone	Ask the patient to relax and let you take the weight of the limb.
	Test shoulder, elbow, wrist and supinator catch; isolate each joint in turn:
	• Hypotonic (hard to detect).
	• Normal.

Tone *(continued)*	• Hypertonic: either:
	  ○ spasticity: velocity-dependent hypertonicity; 'clasp knife': gives way suddenly after initial resistance; UMN, also known as 'pyramidal.'
	  ○ rigidity: stiff throughout the range of movement, like 'bending a lead pipe.' Indicates an 'extrapyramidal' lesion.
	• Cogwheeling: elicited at the wrist, due to a combination of tremor and rigidity (characteristic of Parkinsonism).

Power	MRC scale 0–5. Start proximally and isolate each joint. When describing weakness, think in terms of: • Proximal versus distal. • Unilateral versus bilateral.

MRC power scale

5/5: normal power against resistance.

4/5: reduced power against resistance.

3/5: full range of movement against gravity but none against resistance.

2/5: full range of movement with gravity eliminated.

1/5: flicker of movement.

0/5: no movement.

Reflexes	Hold the tendon hammer at the end and let it fall in a fluid movement. If unable to elicit a reflex, try with reinforcement ('*Clench your teeth*').
	Look at the muscle belly when testing a reflex.
	Record as 'normal,' 'hyper-reflexic' or 'absent' (or 'slow relaxing' in hypothyroidism) (Fig. 6.1).

Reflex	Root	Nerve
Biceps	C5, C6	Musculocutaneous
Supinator	C6, C7	Radial
Triceps	C7, C8	Radial

Figure 6.1 Testing the biceps and triceps reflexes: place your non-dominant hand around the patient's elbow with your thumb over the biceps tendon and your middle finger over the triceps tendon. Strike your thumb and middle finger with a tendon hammer to elicit the biceps and triceps reflexes, respectively.

Coordination	Tests cerebellar function: <ul><li>'Finger–nose test': look for dysmetria and intention tremor.</li><li>Alternating hand-clapping test: look for dysdiadochokinesis.</li><li>Omit if the upper limbs are weak as this will confound the test.</li></ul>
Sensation	Test distally to proximally. Look for 'glove' (length-dependent) or dermatomal loss. There is no need for the patient to close his or her eyes except for proprioception testing. <ul><li>Light touch with fingers (tests spinothalamic pathway):<ul><li>test rapidly by running fingers up the upper limbs (look for 'glove' deficit), then work downwards testing dermatomes, as per Figure 6.2.</li><li>if a deficit is detected, consider refining it by testing pinprick and temperature sensation (also spinothalamic).</li></ul></li><li>Proprioception (i.e. joint position sense, tests dorsal columns): ask the patient to close his or her eyes. Hold the joint at the sides, rather than on the top and bottom, to avoid pressure sensation confounding the test.</li></ul>

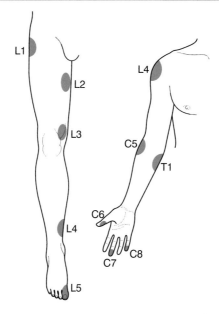

Figure 6.2 Locations to test upper and lower limb dermatomes.

Sensation	If a deficit is detected distally, work
(continued)	proximally to find the most distal
	unaffected joint.
	Consider testing vibration sense (also
	dorsal columns).

Closure	<ul><li>Thank the patient.</li><li>Make sure the patient is comfortable and clothed.</li><li>Wash your hands.</li></ul>Put your findings together: what is the anatomical site of the lesion (LMN *vs.* UMN, pyramidal *vs.* extrapyramidal, etc.?)

TO FINISH

If relevant to findings so far:

Ask the patient to hold his or her upper limbs in front of the body and to close the eyes. Look for:

- Cerebellar dysmetria (on pushing hands down, an 'oscillatory' attempt to return the upper limbs to the neutral position occurs).
- Pronator drift (UMN weakness).
- Pseudoathetosis (proprioceptive loss).

Offer to examine the neurology of the lower limbs and the cranial nerves.

LOWER LIMB EXAMINATION

TO START

WIPE:

Wash your hands.

Introduce yourself to the patient.

Permission: ask to examine the patient.

Position: patient is lying down with lower limbs straight out on the bed.

Pain: check that the patient has no pain.

Exposure: both lower limbs from hips to toes (keep underwear on).

End of the bed	As in the upper limb exam; look for wasting and fasciculation, especially quadriceps and tibialis anterior.
Tone	Ask the patient to relax: • 'Pastry roll' each lower limb and look for 'lag' at the ankle (if not present and the ankle moves in time with the rest of the leg, then tone is increased). • Lift the knee suddenly; the heel lifts off the bed if tone is increased. • Ankle clonus (>5 beats is abnormal; test with knee in flexion). Possible findings: normal, hypertonic (spastic/rigid), reduced, as per upper limb exam.

Movement	Primary muscle[a]	Root	Nerve
Hip flexion	Iliopsoas	L1, L2	Femoral
Hip extension	Gluteus maximus	L5, S1	Inferior gluteal
Knee extension	Quadriceps	L3, L4	Femoral
Knee flexion	Hamstrings	S1	Sciatic
Ankle dorsiflexion	Tibialis anterior	L4	Deep peroneal
Ankle plantar flexion	Gastrocnemius	S1, S2	Tibial
Great toe extension	Extensor hallucis longus	L5	Deep peroneal

[a] Other muscles may also contribute.

Power	MRC scale (see page 48).
	Start proximally and isolate each joint. When describing weakness, think in terms of:
	• Proximal versus distal.
	• Unilateral versus bilateral.
Reflexes	• Hold the tendon hammer at the end and let it fall in a fluid movement.
	• If unable to elicit a reflex, try with reinforcement: Jendrassik manoeuvre (patient interlocks his or her fingers, then pulls).
	• Look at the muscle belly when testing a reflex.
	• Plantar reflex (Fig. 6.3).

Reflexes (continued)	Record as 'normal,' 'hyper-reflexic' or 'absent' (or 'slow relaxing' in hypothyroidism).

Reflex	Root	Nerve
Patellar	L3, L4	Femoral
Ankle	S1, S2	Tibial
Plantar	Upgoing (UMN lesion). Downgoing (normal), absent.	

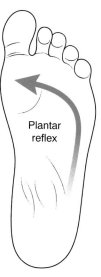

Plantar reflex

Figure 6.3 Testing the plantar reflex: using your thumb nail, apply firm pressure and move swiftly up the lateral border of the patient's foot and across the ball of the foot; watch closely for whether the toes first flex or extend. Flexion is normal, extension is abnormal.

Coordination	Tests cerebellar function:
	• 'Heel–shin test': look for dysmetria.
	• Ask the patient to tap a foot: look for dysdiadochokinesis.
	• Omit if lower limbs are weak as will confound the test.
Sensation	Test distally to proximally. Look for 'glove' (length-dependent) or dermatomal loss. There is no need for the patient to close his or her eyes except for proprioception testing.
	• Light touch with fingers (tests spinothalamic pathway):
	○ test rapidly by running fingers up the lower limbs +/− abdomen (look for 'stocking' deficit or sensory level), then work downwards testing dermatomes, as per Figure 6.2.
	○ if a deficit is detected, consider refining it by testing pinprick and temperature sensation (also spinothalamic).
	• Proprioception (i.e. joint position sense, tests dorsal columns):
	○ ask the patient to close his or her eyes. Hold the joint at the sides, rather than on the top and bottom, to avoid pressure sensation confounding the test.

Sensation *(continued)*	○ if a deficit is detected distally, work proximally to find the most distal unaffected joint. Consider testing vibration sense (also dorsal columns).
Closure	• Thank the patient. • Make sure the patient is comfortable and clothed. • Wash your hands. Put your findings together: what is the anatomical site of the lesion? (LMN *vs.* UMN, pyramidal *vs.* extrapyramidal, etc.)?

Pattern of findings in UMN versus LMN lesions

	UMN	LMN
Inspection	Decorticate posture	Wasting after 2–3 weeks
Tone	Increased +/– clonus	Decreased
Power	Weakness (pyramidal pattern if cortical lesion)	Weakness in distribution of nerve(s)/root(s)/muscle group(s)
Reflexes	Hyper-reflexic, upgoing plantars	Hyporeflexic, downgoing/absent plantars

TO FINISH

If relevant to findings so far:

Ask the patient to walk away, turn, and walk back; observe the gait:

- Ataxia (cerebellar, proprioceptive).
- 'Scissoring' (spasticity).
- Festination, loss of arm swing (Parkinsonism).
- Variable or abnormal stride length or gait width.
- 'Heel–toe walking': ataxia.

Romberg's test (proprioceptive deficit).

Anatomical correctness

NB – The lay terms *arm* and *leg* are used anatomically to indicate the forearm and the lower limb below the knee (as opposed to the upper arm and the thigh, respectively). *Upper limb* and *lower limb* are the correct terms to use for the limbs as a whole.

Chapter 7

Examination of the Breast

TO START	
WIPE:	
Wash your hands.	
Introduce yourself to the patient.	
Permission: ask to examine the patient (a chaperone is advisable and must always be offered).	
Position: start with the patient sitting on the bed with legs hanging over the edge for inspection, then reposition the patient to be lying at 45° for palpation.	
Pain: check that the patient has no pain.	
Exposure: completely exposed from the waist upwards, while ensuring patient privacy.	
End of the bed	Surroundings
	• Observations.
	• Pre-/postoperative management: IV access, IV fluids, drains, catheter, PCA.

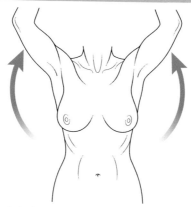

Figure 7.1 Ask the patient to raise her arms slowly out to the side and above her head. This makes tethering of lumps more apparent.

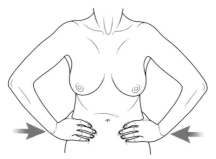

Figure 7.2 Ask the patient to press her hands firmly into her hips; this tenses the pectoral muscles. Observe for the appearance, or disappearance, of lumps, indicating if they are superficial or deep to the muscle.

Palpation	Position the patient at 45° with one hand behind the head on the side being examined, thus spreading the breast tissue and making it easier to appreciate a mass.
	Breast Examine the 'normal' breast before the 'abnormal' breast: • Palpate the whole breast with the flats of the fingers in a methodical fashion. • The borders of the breast are the clavicle (superiorly), the sternum (medially), the bra strap line (inferiorly) and the midaxillary line (laterally). • Methodical approaches include concentric circles starting at the nipple and spiralling outwards until the axillary tail or palpating each of the four quadrants, the nipple and the axillary tail. • If nipple inversion is noted, attempt eversion or ask the patient to attempt to do so.

Palpation (continued)	If a lump is found:

Lump

Using both hands, ascertain:

- Site: left or right breast and quadrant.
- Size: normally quantitative and in two dimensions.
- Shape: may be regular (e.g. round or oval) or irregular.
- Surface: smooth or irregular.
- Edge: distinct or indistinct.
- Consistency: soft, firm, rubbery, or stony hard.
- Mobility, fixation, and tethering: indicates attachment to underlying and overlying structures.
- Tenderness.

Common breast lumps

- Carcinoma tends to occur in older women and commonly presents with an irregular, stony hard, painless lump that is tethered or fixed.
- Fibroadenoma tends to occur in younger women and commonly presents with a smooth, rubbery, painless lump that is highly mobile.
- Breast cysts tend to occur in older women and commonly present with a smooth, soft, mobile lump that may be painful.
- Fibroadenosis affects women of any age and presents with indistinct 'lumpiness' of the breast tissue that often varies with the menstrual cycle and may be painful.

Palpation (continued)	Axilla
	Take the weight of the patient's arm by resting it on your shoulder or supporting the patient's forearm with your other hand (relaxes the pectoral muscles).
	Examine the 'normal' side before the 'abnormal' side:
	• Warn the patient that palpation may be painful, particularly in the apex.
	• Use the right hand to palpate the left axilla and the left hand to palpate the right axilla.
	• Palpate the three sides of the axillary pyramid (medial, posterior and lateral) and the apex using the flats of the fingers.
	• Repeat on the abnormal side and compare: small bilateral lymph nodes may be normal; enlarged unilateral, rubbery, hard lymph nodes may indicate underlying malignancy.
	• If axillary lymphadenopathy is found, palpate supraclavicular and cervical lymph nodes.
Closure	• Thank the patient.
	• Leave the patient to get dressed in privacy.
	• Wash your hands.

TO FINISH

If relevant to findings so far:

Examinations

Examination of the abdomen: hepatomegaly and ascites with liver metastases.

Examination of the spine: bony tenderness, restricted movements, and limited straight leg raise with bony metastases.

Examination of the lung bases: pleural effusions with lung metastases.

Examination of the arms: lymphoedema with obstructed lymphatics.

Investigations

Ultrasound or mammogram.

FNA of the lump.

Chapter 8

Examination of the Skin

TO START

WIPE

Wash hands.

Introduce yourself.

Permission: ask to examine the patient.

Position: including adequate lighting.

Pain: ask whether a lump/skin lesion is painful.

Exposure: of the affected region and the contralateral side.

Inspection	Location
	• Distance of a lump from the nearest bony prominence.
	• Is the problem localised or generalised?
	Size
	On inspection; for a lump, this will be confirmed later on palpation.

Inspection *(continued)*	Shape
	Appearance of overlying skin:
	• Erythema.
	• Pigmentation.
	• Punctum.
	• Ulceration/necrosis.
	• Excoriations.
	• Blistering or pustules.
	• Scaling.
	• Scars.
Palpation	Overlying skin
	• Smooth or rough?
	• Is the lesion flat or raised?
	• Is there scaling (implies involvement of the epidermis)?
	Temperature
	With the back of your hand, compare the temperature of the affected area with the same area on the contralateral side.
	Size
	Use a tape measure for more superficial lumps or skin lesions so that growth can be objectively monitored in the future.
	• General impression for deeper lumps.
	• Length and width.
	Shape
	• Consider in three dimensions (i.e. 'spherical,' etc.).

Palpation
(continued)
	• Are the margins discrete or not?
	
	Consistency
	• Soft (benign)?
	• Rubbery (lymph node)?
	• Hard (bony or neoplastic)?
	• Pulsatile?
	• Attempt to distinguish whether pulsatility is arising from the lump or from an adjacent vessel.
	• If intrinsic to the lump, is it expansile as well as pulsatile (aneurysm)?
	
	Mobility
	• Test in two directions: is it mobile, fixed or tethered (overlying skin puckers as lump is moved)?
	• Test with underlying muscle relaxed and contracted:
	  ○ contraction renders a mobile lump fixed; indicates muscle infiltration.
	  ○ contraction renders a palpable lump impalpable; indicates lump is deep to the muscle.
	
	Reducibility
	• A *reducible* lump will disappear with pressure and will not return spontaneously (e.g. a hernia).

Palpation *(continued)*	• *Compressible* lumps disappear/ decrease in size with pressure but reappear spontaneously (e.g. saphena varix). Fluctuance Place two fingers on either side of the lesion and feel for protrusion while applying pressure to the lump with another finger. Fluctuance implies a fluid-filled or fatty lump. Transillumination Shine a pen torch across the lump, either in a dark room or while shielding the lump with your other hand to block external light. A lump containing clear fluid, such as a cystic lesion, will transilluminate (note: a lipoma may also transilluminate).
Percussion	Gas-filled lumps will be resonant (e.g. a hernia of a loop of bowel).
Auscultation	• BS (e.g. a hernia). • Bruits or murmurs may be heard in vascular lesions or lumps with increased blood supply.
Closure	• Thank the patient. • Make sure the patient is comfortable and clothed. • Wash your hands.

TO FINISH

- Assess the regional lymph nodes draining the lump/lesion.
- For skin lesions, consider examining the scalp, nails and mucosal surfaces (mouth, eyes and genital region) for involvement.
- Look at observations, including temperature, if considering an inflammatory/infectious lesion.
- Look for evidence of weight loss, or record BMI, as a sign of malignancy.
- Consider further examination of skin lesions with a dermatoscope if trained to do so.

Examination of the Hand

WIPE
Wash your hands.
Introduce yourself to the patient.
Permission: ask to examine the patient.
Position: start with the patient placing his or her hands (palm down) on a pillow.
Pain: check that the patient has no pain.
Exposure: expose the arms to above the elbow.

Inspection (hands and elbows)	Examine the dorsal aspect, then volar.
	Skin
	• Scars: carpal tunnel release, joint replacements.
	• Texture: tight, thickened, shiny (systemic sclerosis), thinning (steroid use).

| Inspection (hands and elbows) *(continued)* | • Rash: finger-pulp infarct (vasculitis), silvery scale (psoriasis), violaceous papules (also known as Gottron's papules [dermatomyositis]).
• Colour: white, blue or red fingertips (Raynaud's syndrome).

Nails
• Onycholysis, pitting, longitudinal ridges (psoriasis).
• Nailfold infarcts (vasculitis).
• Dilated nailfold capillaries (systemic sclerosis, dermatomyositis).

Soft tissue
• Muscle wasting.
• Soft tissue swellings: rheumatoid nodules (extensor aspect of elbow), ganglia.
• Subcutaneous deposits: calcinosis of finger pulps (limited cutaneous systemic sclerosis), subcutaneous deposits around joints (gouty tophi).

Joints and bones
• Deformities.
• Rheumatoid arthritis: Z-shaped thumb, Boutonnière's deformity, mallet finger, swan necking, MCP ulnar deviation, radial deviation of the wrist. |

Inspection (hands and elbows) (continued)	• Osteoarthritis: Heberden's nodes (distal IPJs), Bouchard's nodes (proximal IPJs).
Palpation	Skin • Temperature. • Radial pulse. • Sensation: median nerve (thenar eminence), ulnar nerve (hypothenar eminence), radial nerve (dorsum of first web space). Soft tissue • Thenar and hypothenar eminences: wasting. • Tendons: thickening or nodularity. • Swellings (e.g. rheumatoid nodules). Joints • Note swelling, temperature, discomfort. • Wrist joint: examine with two thumbs on the extensor surface and index fingers on the flexor surface. • Each MCP joint, each IPJ: hold between finger and index finger, squeezing each joint in turn. • Elbow joint.
Movement	Assess active and passive movement of each joint in isolation.

Movement (continued)	• Wrist:
	  o flexion and extension.
	• Fingers:
	  o extension and flexion of MCP and IPJs.
	  o abduction and adduction of MCP joints.
	• Thumb:
	  o abduction: point the thumb upwards, maintain against resistance.
	  o opposition: hold the thumb to each fingertip, maintain against resistance.

Functional assessment	Ask the patient to demonstrate: • Power grip: grip around the middle and index fingers and squeeze. • Pincer grip: hold a key or piece of paper between thumb and index finger. • Precision grip: the patient forms a ring with their thumb and forefinger, whilst the examiner attempts to break the ring with one of their own fingers (Fig. 9.1). • Daily tasks (e.g. undo button, pick up a coin, hold a pen).

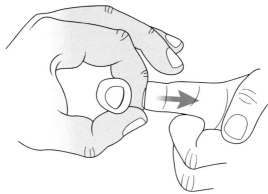

Figure 9.1 Precision grip: ask the patient to make a ring with their index finger and thumb. Try to break this circle using your hooked index finger.

Special tests	Phalen's test
	Forced flexion of the wrist against the other hand re-creates carpal tunnel symptoms.
	Tinel's test
	Percussion over the median nerve on the volar aspect of the wrist reproduces paraesthesia in the median nerve distribution and is a sign of carpal tunnel syndrome.

Special tests (continued)	Froment's test
	Ask the patient to hold a piece of paper between thumb and index finger; attempt to pull the paper away. This detects ulnar nerve palsy. With an intact ulnar nerve, the IPJ of the thumb is extended, and grip is maintained through the action of adductor pollicis. In ulnar nerve palsy, the action of adductor pollicis is lost, and the grip must be maintained by flexor pollicis longus. This results in flexion at the IPJ of the thumb (Froment's test positive).
Closure	• Thank the patient. • Make sure the patient is comfortable and clothed. • Wash your hands.

Remember Heberden's nodes affect the distal IPJs. They are the 'outer Hebrides.'

Chapter 10

Examination of the Shoulder

Examination of the shoulder, like any joint, must follow the 'look, feel, move' principles. Always ask the patient which is the affected side and examine the normal joint first. Comparing both sides is essential to detect pathology.

TO START

WIPE:

Wash your hands.

Introduce yourself to the patient.

Permission: ask to examine the patient.

Position: start with the patient standing.

Pain: check that the patient has no pain.

Exposure: remove top (women can keep their bra on).

End of the bed	• Assess gait on walking into the room: is there a clue to the diagnosis that affects other joints?
	• Posture: is the patient in a comfortable and neutral position?

End of the bed *(continued)*	• Is the patient using a sling? • Is the patient using a walking aid?
Look	Always remember to compare both sides. Observe from the front, side and back. Skin • Erythema. • Scars. • Sinuses. Soft tissue • Muscle wasting: deltoids, biceps, supra- and infraspinatus. • Swelling of joints. Bones and joints • Asymmetry • Visible deformity at the sternoclavicular, acromioclavicular or glenohumeral joints.
Feel	Always check if or where the patient is experiencing pain. Skin • Tenderness. • Temperature. Soft tissue • Assess muscle bulk and tenderness: trapezius, deltoids, biceps, supra- and infraspinatus.

Feel *(continued)*	Bones and joints • Feel sternoclavicular joint and work along the clavicle to the acromioclavicular joint. • Feel the acromion and along the spine of the scapula. • Feel the anterior and posterior joint lines and the glenohumeral joint.
Move	Always assess both active and passive movements. Active • Flexion: normal limit of movement: 165°. • Extension. • Abduction: normal limit of movement 180°. • External rotation: normal limit of movement 60°. • Internal rotation: assess how far the patient can reach up his or her back. Passive Repeat all movements passively; feel for any crepitus or resistance.
Special tests	Ask the patient to push against a wall and look for winging of the scapula. This implies serratus anterior paralysis, seen in long thoracic nerve damage.

Special tests *(continued)*	**Impingement test** Abduct the shoulder to 90° with the elbow fully extended and the thumbs pointing downwards and the arms slightly forwards (in the plane of the scapula). Push down on the arm and check for pain. **Apprehension test** The shoulder is abducted to 90°, the elbow flexed to 90° and the forearm straight up in the air. Place one hand over the scapula and the other on the forearm. Using the forearm as a lever, forcibly externally rotate the shoulder whilst pushing anteriorly on the scapula. Apprehension during this test implies shoulder joint instability. **Scarf test** Place the patient's hand on the contralateral shoulder, with the elbow of the active arm raised level with the chin. Apply pressure to the elbow to push the hand posteriorly. Pain during this test indicates dysfunction of the acromioclavicular joint.
Closure	• Thank the patient. • Make sure the patient is comfortable and clothed. • Wash your hands.

TO FINISH

- Assess the joint above and below: i.e. neck and elbow. Pathology at these joints can refer pain to the shoulder.

- Perform a full neurovascular examination of the upper limbs.

- Request imaging as indicated.

Chapter 11

Examination of the Hip

Examination of the hip, like any joint, must follow the 'look, feel, move' principles. Always ask the patient which is the affected side and examine the normal joint first. Comparing both sides is essential to detect pathology.

TO START

WIPE

Wash your hands.

Introduce yourself to the patient.

Permission: ask to examine the patient; explain that the examination may cause discomfort.

Position: start with the patient standing; the patient will need to lie down later.

Pain: check that the patient has no pain.

Exposure: both knees should be visible; the patient should ideally be undressed to their underwear.

Look	Standing • Muscle wasting: particularly gluteal muscle bulk.

Look *(continued)*	Supine • Fixed flexion deformity. • Scars. • Leg length discrepancy: to measure true leg length, use a tape measure from the anterior superior iliac spine to the medial malleolus; a difference >1 cm is significant. ○ fractured neck of femur classically presents with a shortened and externally rotated leg.
Feel	Greater trochanter tenderness: bursitis, gluteus medius tendonitis.
Move	Supine • Flexion (with knee flexed to 90°): normal range of movement 120–135°. • Abduction: 40–50°. • Adduction: 20–30°. Prone • Extension: 20–30°. • Internal rotation (with knee flexed to 90°): 30°. • External rotation (with knee flexed to 90°): 50°. Gait • Antalgic (painful): nonspecific. • Trendelenburg (lateral lean on weight-bearing side): gluteus medius weakness.

Move (continued)	• Lurching with posterior lean: gluteus maximus weakness.

Overview of innervation at the hip

Nerve	Root	Sensory	Motor
Genitofemoral	L1–2	Proximal anteromedial thigh	
Obturator	L2–4	Inferomedial thigh	Hip adduction
Lateral femoral cutaneous	L2–3	Lateral thigh	
Femoral	L2–4	Anteromedial thigh	Hip flexion Knee extension
Superior gluteal	L5		Hip abduction
Inferior gluteal	L5–S2		Hip extension
Sciatic	L4–S2		Knee flexion
Posterior femoral cutaneous	S1–3	Posterior thigh	

Special tests	Thomas's test
	To assess for fixed flexion deformity of the hip: place your hand under the lumbar spine to immobilise, then fully flex one hip and observe the opposite leg. If the opposite leg lifts off the couch, then there is fixed flexion deformity of that hip.

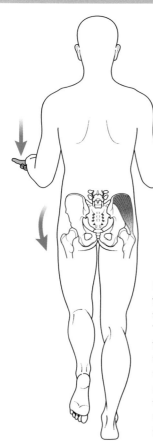

Figure 11.1 Trendelenburg test. Stand facing the patient with their hands on yours. The patient stands on one leg then the other. Hip abductor weakness in the standing leg will cause the unsupported side of the pelvis to drop and the patient will press down with the contralateral hand to steady themselves.

Special tests *(continued)*	Trendelenburg test To assess for gluteal weakness: ask the patient to stand on one leg; the pelvis should remain level. However, if the test is positive, the pelvis will dip on the contralateral side (Fig. 11.1). Femoroacetabular impingement Pain on sequential flexion, adduction and internal rotation. Hip instability In infants, perform Barlow's test (dislocation: hips at 90° and adducted with downward pressure) and Ortolani's test (reduction: hips at 90° and gently abducted) to identify hip instability.
Closure	• Thank the patient. • Make sure the patient is comfortable and clothed. • Wash your hands.

TO FINISH

• Examine the knee joint; pathology here can refer pain to the hip.

• Perform a neurovascular examination.

• Request AP and lateral (cross-table) X-rays if appropriate.

Chapter 12

Examination of the Knee

Examination of the knee, like any joint, must follow the 'look, feel, move' principles. Always ask the patient which is the affected side and examine the normal joint first. Comparing both sides is essential to detect pathology.

TO START

WIPE:

Wash your hands.

Introduce yourself to the patient.

Permission: ask to examine the patient; explain that the examination may cause discomfort.

Position: start with the patient standing; the patient will need to lie down later.

Pain: check that the patient has no pain.

Exposure: both knees should be visible; the patient ideally should be undressed to their underwear.

EXAMINATION IN THE STANDING POSITION

Look | Can the patient stand straight with the feet together? Is this limited by pain or deformity?

Skin changes
Look anteriorly (A) and posteriorly (P): eczema (P), psoriatic plaques (A), erythema (A and P), popliteal swellings (P), scars (A and P).

Alignment
Alignment is normal when the patella is pointing forwards when viewed from the front and the femoral condyles and medial malleoli touch.
- Genu varum: femoral condyles are wide apart when the feet are together (e.g. medial compartment OA or normal variant).
- Genu valgum: femoral condyles touch, resulting in an increased intermalleolar distance (e.g. lateral compartment OA or normal variant).

Intercondylar and intermalleolar distances can be measured in centimetres.

Wasting
Underuse, neurological lesions (e.g. lower motor neuron lesion), malnutrition.

Look (continued)	Hypertrophy
	Exercise, drugs (steroids), metabolic (e.g. Duchenne muscular dystrophy).
Feel	Muscle bulk: wasting or hypertrophy of the quadriceps (particularly vastus medialis) can be observed and measured by measuring the circumference of the quadriceps 10 cm superior to the tibial tuberosity and comparing both sides.
Move	Walk the patient to the end of the bed: do they have a limp?

EXAMINATION IN THE LYING POSITION

Look	Deformity such as a fixed flexion, erythema, scars (due to surgery or trauma), swollen knee, dermatological changes: <ul><li>Fixed flexion deformity is seen in severe OA.</li><li>Total knee replacement scars are in the midline, over the patella.</li><li>Arthroscopy scars are 1-cm incisions around the knee joint.</li></ul>
Feel	<ul><li>Temperature.</li></ul> For an effusion (e.g. septic, osteo-, rheumatoid or crystal arthrithides, or post-traumatic): <ul><li>Crepitus.</li></ul>

| **Feel**
(continued) | • 'Patellar tap test': a large effusion will cause the patella to 'bounce' when pushed down.
• 'Stroke test'. |

The 'stroke test'
'Milk' the fluid from the suprapatellar compartment with one hand to 'fill' the knee. Keep this hand over the suprapatellar compartment and with the other hand stroke the medial compartment of the knee to empty fluid into the lateral compartment. A bulge in the lateral compartment indicates an effusion.

Place your hand on the extended knee and ask the patient to flex to 90°. Then, palpate systematically:
• Medial collateral ligaments.
• Medial femoral condyle.
• Medial patellar border (tender in anterior knee pain syndrome).
• Lateral femoral condyle.
• Lateral tibial condyle (lateral joint line of the knee).
• Lateral collateral ligaments.
• Tibial tuberosity (tender in apophysitis [Osgood Schlatter disease]).
• Medial tibial condyle (medial joint line of the knee).

Popliteal fossa
Swelling here may be a Baker's cyst, popliteal aneurysm or DVT.

Move	• Test flexion and extension against resistance: the patient's heel should be off the bed; isolate the knee joint with a hand on the thigh.
	• Move the patella from side to side with the patient's knee extended; pain is felt in patellofemoral compartment in osteoarthritis.
	• Test the collateral ligaments with valgus (MCL) and varus (LCL) stress.
	• Test the cruciate ligaments: hold the knee in flexion, with the thumb on the tibial tuberosity and the rest of the fingers grasping the knee in the popliteal fossa:
	○ anterior draw test: pull anteriorly; laxity indicates ACL instability (Fig. 12.1).

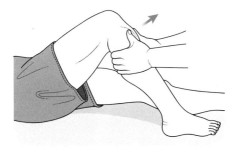

Figure 12.1 Anterior draw test: assesses anterior cruciate ligament instability.

Move *(continued)*	○ posterior draw test: push posteriorly; laxity indicates PCL instability.
Special tests	Patellar apprehension test Tests: patellar dislocation that reduces spontaneously. With the patient lying on the bed, the knee is passively flexed slightly (0–30°); quadriceps is relaxed. The patella is then pushed laterally by the examiner. Often, patients do not like this test. McMurray's test Tests: meniscal tears (Fig. 12.2). With one hand, hold the flexed knee along the joint line and provide a valgus stress (hand on the lateral side of the knee). The other hand holds the foot and externally rotates the leg whilst extending the knee. Pain or a 'click' indicates a tear in the medial meniscus. Repeating this but internally rotating the leg in extension with a varus stress (hand on the medial side of the knee) will elicit lateral meniscus tears. Apley's grinding test Tests: meniscal tears. The patient is prone and the knee flexed to 90°. The tibia is then compressed onto the knee joint while

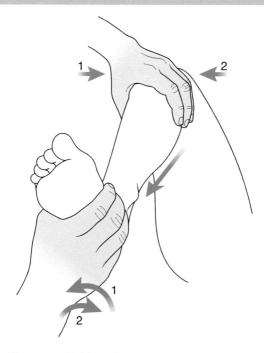

Figure 12.2 McMurray's test.
1. Apply a valgus stress with your hand on the knee joint-line. Extend the knee while externally rotating the leg. Feel and listen for a click.
2. Repeat with a varus stress and internal rotation while extending the knee.

Special tests *(continued)*	externally rotated. Pain elicited signifies meniscal damage. Then, apply traction to pull the tibia from the femur. If rotating the tibia internally and externally elicits pain, this may indicate collateral ligament damage.
Closure	• Thank the patient. • Make sure the patient is comfortable and clothed. • Wash your hands.

TO FINISH

• Examine the hip and ankle joints; pathology here can refer pain to the knee.

• Neurovascular examination.

• Request AP and lateral X-rays.

Chapter 13

Clerking Examination

TO START

WIPE:

Wash your hands.

Introduce yourself to the patient.

Permission: ask to examine the patient.

Position: start with the patient sitting at 45°; lie the patient flat when you come to the abdominal exam.

Pain: check that the patient has no pain.

Exposure: remove top (women can keep their bra on but be careful not to miss an underlying scar); undo the top button of trousers and pull down to the level of the pubic symphysis.

End of the bed	Surroundings
	• Monitoring: ECG (electrocardiogram), observations.
	• Treatments: O$_2$, infusions, vascular access, catheter (urethral or suprapubic), mobility aids.

End of the bed *(continued)*	Patient Sick or well? Alert or drowsy? Short of breath? Complexion: pale (anaemia, hypotension); flushed; jaundiced. Cachexia or obesity? Remarkable odour: alcohol, cigarette smoke, ketosis. Signs of self-neglect? Quickly assess gross neurological function: consciousness level, movement of limbs, speech. Look for tremors, abnormal posturing or facial asymmetry. Any of these findings should indicate including a comprehensive neurological examination in your clerking.
Hands	Are they warm and well-perfused? Nails • Clubbing. • Splinter haemorrhages: trauma or bacterial endocarditis. • CRT: must be examined at or above the level of the heart (<2 s is normal). • Koilonychia: brittle, spoon-shaped nails (chronic iron deficiency). • Leuconychia: white nails (hypoalbuminaemia).

Hands (continued)	• Onycholysis: detachment of the nail from the bed (psoriasis).
	Hands
	• Joints: signs of osteoarthritis (Heberden's nodes: distal IPJs) or rheumatoid arthritis (Bouchard's nodes: proximal IPJs; swan neck deformity; Boutonnière deformity; ulnar deviation at the wrist).
	• Osler's nodes, Janeway lesions: bacterial endocarditis.
	• Pale palmar creases: anaemia.
	• Palmar erythema: chronic liver disease.
	• Tendon xanthomata: familial hypercholesterolaemia.
	• Dupuytren's contracture: idiopathic, occupational, smoking or alcoholic liver disease.
	• Skin turgor: a soft sign of hydration status.
Arms	Radial pulse
	• Rate: count for 15 s, then multiply by 4.
	• Rhythm: regular, regularly irregular or irregularly irregular (atrial fibrillation).

Arms *(continued)*	Wrist Asterixis: a sign of encephalopathy in liver disease or CO_2 retention. Arms Look for: • Track marks (IVDU). • Bruises and excoriations. Measure blood pressure (ideally in both arms).
Face	Characteristic appearance (e.g. mitral facies, cushingoid features, Down syndrome). Eyes • Corneal arcus: normal in the elderly, hyperlipidaemia in young people. • Scleral icterus: jaundice. • Pale conjunctiva: anaemia. • Xanthelasma: hyperlipidaemia. • Thyroid eye disease: exopthalmos, lid retraction, lid lag, conjunctival injection and chemosis. Mouth • Angular stomatitis, glossitis: B_{12}/folate deficiency. • Mouth ulcers: Crohn's disease, coeliac, idiopathic. • Mucous membranes: hydration status.

Face *(continued)*	• Under the tongue: central cyanosis. • Poor dentition: bacterial endocarditis risk.
Neck	Carotid pulse • Volume: normal, high volume, low volume. • Character: normal, collapsing, slow rising. Jugular venous pressure (JVP) Measure with the patient sitting at 45°. Find the vertical distance between the angle of Louis (manubriosternal angle) and the top of the JVP. It is normally <3 cm.
Precordium	Inspection • Respiratory rate. • Chest expansion: check for symmetry and the presence of paradoxical movement in trauma (flail segment). • Shape: pectus carinatum, barrel chest, pectus excavatum, scoliosis or kyphosis. • Stigmata of liver disease: spider naevi, gynaecomastia. • Scars: sternotomy (likely CABG) or valve replacement), posterolateral thoracotomy (e.g. mitral valve surgery), pacemaker (usually below left clavicle).

| **Precordium** *(continued)* | • Radiotherapy stigmata: localisation tattoos or skin changes secondary to radiation.
• Visible apex beat.

Palpation
• Apex: normally in left fifth intercostal space, midclavicular line (often just below the nipple).
• Palpable/impalpable?
• Character: normal, sustained (increased afterload), double impulse (palpable third or fourth heart sound).
• Position: normal, displaced (cardiomegaly).
• Parasternal heave: press firmly to feel for ventricular hypertrophy.
• Thrills: press lightly over base of heart to detect palpable murmurs.

Auscultation
Listen whilst feeling carotid pulse. At each area try to identify:
• First heart sound: AV valves closing.
• Second heart sound: aortic/ pulmonary valves closing.
• Third heart sound: rapid ventricular filling.
• Fourth heart sound: atrial contraction against a non-compliant ventricle. |

Precordium *(continued)*	• Additional sounds: prosthetic valves.
	• Murmurs: listen in systole, listen in diastole.

Diaphragm of stethoscope (high-pitched sounds)
• Apex ('mitral' area).
• Lower left sternal edge ('tricuspid' area).
• Upper left sternal edge ('pulmonary' area).
• Upper right sternal edge ('aortic' area).

If you hear a murmur: track radiation into axilla/carotids.

Bell of stethoscope (low-pitched sounds: press gently)
• Carotid bruits: the patient should hold his or her breath and so should you.
• Apex.

Dynamic manoeuvres: for diastolic murmurs
• With the bell in place over the apex, the patient rolls into the left lateral position with the left hand behind the head. Breath is held in expiration (mitral stenosis).

Precordium *(continued)*	• The patient sits forwards; listen at the lower left sternal edge with the diaphragm. Breath is held in expiration (aortic regurgitation). Palpate for sacral oedema.
Lungs (Part 1)	**With patient still sitting forwards:** Listen to the anterior lung fields.
Neck	Lower the head of the bed until it is horizontal; position yourself behind the patient. Palpate: cervical lymphadenopathy, thyroid.
Lungs (Part 2)	Inspection Scars: thoracotomy, spinal surgery, nephrectomy. Palpation • Expansion: check for equal lateral chest expansion; ask the patient to empty his or her lungs; place your hands around the ribs with your thumbs touching in the midline and ask the patient to take a full breath in. • Tenderness: if the patient has complained of chest pain, palpate for bony tenderness.

Lungs (Part 2) *(continued)*	Percussion Systematically percuss the lung fields, including the axillae, and compare both sides. Auscultation Ask the patient to breathe normally through an open mouth. • Listen in the same points as percussion; compare both sides: crepitations, wheeze, reduced air entry. • Vocal resonance can add more information if any abnormalities are found.
Abdomen	**Lie the patient down flat.** Inspection • Scars, recent surgical wounds, stoma bag, bruising. • Distension: fluid, fat, flatus, faeces, foetus. • Ask the patient to take a deep breath in: peritonism. • Ask the patient to cough: hernias. Palpation Systematically palpate the nine regions of the abdomen, starting furthest from any area of tenderness.

Abdomen (continued)	Watch the patient's face for signs of discomfort. Palpate superficially at first, then deeply. Feel for liver, spleen, kidneys, abdominal aorta, distended bladder.
	Percussion Liver, spleen, bladder, ascites (shifting dullness).
	Auscultation • Listen for BS: normal, high pitched, absent. • Listen for bruits in the abdominal aorta and over the renal arteries bilaterally.
Legs	• Palpate for pitting oedema. • Glance at the feet (e.g. clubbing, signs of embolism). • Test the plantar reflexes as an absolute minimum.

NB – If you clinically suspect neurological pathology or the following examinations are abnormal, you must perform a full neurological assessment (see the relevant chapters).

Gross neurological assessment	Cranial nerves • 'Follow my finger with your eyes': III/ IV/VI, nystagmus. • 'Raise your eyebrows', 'Shut your eyes', 'Show me your teeth': VII. • 'Stick out your tongue': XII.

Gross neurological assessment *(continued)*	Upper limbs • *'Raise your arms up'*. • *'Wiggle your fingers'*. • *'Turn your palms face up; close your eyes'*: pronator drift. Lower limbs • *'Wiggle your toes'*. • Test plantar reflexes.
Closure	• Thank the patient. • Make sure the patient is comfortable and clothed. • Wash your hands.

TO FINISH

If relevant to findings so far:

Examinations

Complete examination of the upper and lower limb neurology and the cranial nerves.

Examine the patient's gait.

Focused examination of any skin lesions, rashes, lumps or joint pathology.

Bedside tests

ECG.

A full set of observations.

Urine dipstick, including β-hCG for females of reproductive age.

TO FINISH (continued)

Investigations

Chest X-ray.

Abdominal X-ray if indicated.

Bloods (exact tests depend on differential diagnosis; however, full blood count, U&Es, CRP and liver function tests are a good starting point).

Chapter 14

Presenting Your Findings

Presenting your findings can be the most difficult part of clerking and takes lots of practice. It is also your chance to shine and show that you are thinking rather than just regurgitating your history and examination findings verbatim. A good presentation should be delivered like a well-structured argument that sweeps towards a foregone conclusion: your differential diagnosis. You must formulate your differential before you present. Then, you can 'build a case' for it by offering supporting evidence from the history and examination. Of course, one must not go too far; it is important to include relevant information even if it makes your chosen diagnosis less likely. **Concision**, **clarity** and **structure** are key. Be prepared to adapt your style to your consultant; some value brevity, and others prefer a more comprehensive, traditionally structured presentation. What follows are simply pieces of advice; you must find your own voice.

Here are a few pointers to get you started:

1. Stay calm.

2. Do not fiddle. Take off your stethoscope and hold it with both hands behind your back, this looks neat and stops you pointing at parts of your own body while presenting.

3. Look at the consultant, not the patient, when you present.

4. Be clear, confident and definite about what you have found (e.g. '*On auscultation, there were coarse crepitations at the right base*' versus '*I think there might have been some crackles on the right.*').

5. Do not recount your entire clerking; you have documented it in the notes. Only present positive and significant negative findings. The clinician to whom you are presenting can always ask for more detail should it be required.

6. Normal findings should only be presented if their normality is unexpected in the context of your other abnormal findings. In other situations, a normal finding is inconsequential. For example, a soft, non-tender abdomen in a patient with a cough is not important, but in someone with bloody diarrhoea, it is highly relevant.

7. 'Err' and 'umm' are not medical terms.

THE PRESENTATION

Introduce the patient	Name, age and occupation if relevant: *'The next patient is Mr X, a 54-year-old truck driver.'*
Provide context for the presentation	This is a synthesis of relevant past medical history, risk factors and functional status or premorbid condition: *'Mr X is a current smoker with a 30-pack-year history; he has known hypercholesterolaemia and was diagnosed with type 2 diabetes 4 years ago, for which he takes metformin.'*
State the presenting complaint	Give a brief history of the events leading to admission. Include important negative findings to clarify your suspected diagnosis after you have listed the symptoms that the patient has experienced: *'Mr X presents with crushing central chest pain that radiates into the left arm. The pain began 2 hours ago at rest; he initially rated it as 8 out of 10, but it has responded to sublingual GTN and IV morphine on arrival at hospital. He has not been nauseous or sweaty and the pain is not pleuritic.'*

Give the relevant past medical history	Mention important related conditions from which the patient does not suffer: 'Mr X is a type 2 diabetic but otherwise has no past medical history; of note, he has no history of ischaemic heart disease.'
Give the drug history	If the patient has a true drug allergy, be sure to mention it. It is usually unnecessary to specify doses and timings of medications, although these should definitely be documented in your written clerking: . 'He takes simvastatin and metformin.'
Present any relevant family and social history	Smoking and alcohol intake should always be included. A patient's functional status and living situation are important when it comes to discharge planning but consider whether they are relevant to your presentation of an acute admission to hospital. Exercise tolerance is also useful, especially if there has been a recent change: 'There is no strong family history of cardiovascular disease. He drinks 25 units a week, lives with his wife, and is independent.' (Smoking was mentioned at the beginning of the presentation, so we do not need to repeat it here.)

Present your examination findings	If the examination is normal, simply say so and move on:
	'The examination is entirely unremarkable, and the observations are stable.'
	Otherwise, present any abnormal examination findings in the order that you would have detected them. Also, include any findings that are normal as long as their normality informs your differential diagnosis (i.e. they help you to exclude other possible diagnoses with a similar history).
	'On examination, Mr X appears anxious and is short of breath at rest. He is tachycardic with a pulse of 120 bpm and tachypnoeic with a respiratory rate of 25 breaths/min. His peripheries are cool, and his CRT is 3 seconds. On auscultation, there is a pansystolic murmur, heard loudest at the apex and radiating to the axilla. There is no radioradial difference; the blood pressures in each arm are equal, and there is no chest wall tenderness on palpation.'

Present your examination findings *(continued)*	Give the details of any investigations that have been performed so far:
	'The ECG shows ST segment depression in the lateral chest leads. The chest X-ray and blood results are normal; of note, the initial troponin is negative.'
	Summarise the case in a few key sentences:
	'In summary, this 54-year-old gentleman presents with a 2-hour history of cardiac-sounding chest pain on a background of type 2 diabetes and a strong smoking history. He shows signs of shock and a murmur consistent with mitral regurgitation. The ECG demonstrates lateral ST depression.'
Give your differential diagnosis and initial management	*'My top differential diagnosis for this gentleman's chest pain would be an ACS. This is supported by the ST depression seen on ECG. I have started the ACS protocol. We are completing a set of serial ECGs and will send a 12-hour troponin. Other differentials include musculoskeletal chest pain, although there is no chest wall tenderness, and pulmonary embolism; however, there are no signs of a deep venous thrombosis, and the chest pain is not of a pleuritic nature.'*

OTHER EXAMPLE PRESENTATIONS

'Mrs Y. is an 88-year-old lady who was admitted from her nursing home this morning. She has a background of COPD and heart failure; she has oxygen at the nursing home and is normally hoisted between bed and chair. She presents with a 3-day history of cough, productive of green sputum, worsening shortness of breath and reduced oral intake. Her GP started her on amoxicillin and 30 mg prednisolone yesterday. Mrs Y. normally takes inhalers and antihypertensives as listed here. On examination, she is requiring 35% oxygen to maintain saturations of 90%; she is tachypnoeic at a rate of 24 bpm and is using her accessory muscles of respiration. Her temperature on admission was 38.4°C. Auscultation of the chest reveals bibasal crepitations, worse on the left, and global expiratory wheeze. There is an associated increase in vocal resonance on the left side of the chest. There is significant dependent oedema evident bilaterally up to the knees. The chest X-ray shows cardiomegaly, blunting of both costophrenic angles and left lower zone consolidation. Her arterial blood gas on 35% O_2 showed a partially compensated respiratory acidosis with a pH of 7.34, pO_2 of 8.5, pCO_2 of 7 and a base excess of -4. In summary, this 88-year-old lady presents pyrexial with a productive cough on a background of COPD and heart failure with X-ray changes consistent with a left lower lobe pneumonia. My leading differential diagnosis is a pneumonia causing an infective exacerbation of COPD; I have sent bloods for analysis, including blood cultures, and I have started antibiotics, steroids, nebulisers and fluids as per the hospital guidelines.'

'Mr Z. is a 63-year-old gentleman who has had several recent admissions under the gastroenterologists for upper GI bleeding. Mr Z. drinks one and a half bottles of wine daily; has oesophageal varices, which were recently banded; and cirrhosis of the liver on a recent abdominal ultrasound. He presents with a 1-week history of worsening abdominal distension and associated shortness of breath; in the last 24 hours, he has become febrile and complains of rigors. Mr Z.'s other significant past medical history includes a myocardial infarct 2 years ago with subsequent angioplasty and type 2 diabetes. He takes metformin, aspirin, vitamin supplements, an angiotensin-converting enzyme inhibitor and a statin. He has an anaphylactic reaction to penicillin. On examination, Mr Z. is disoriented to time and place; he has a coarse tremor and demonstrable asterixis. He has marked palmar erythema, multiple bruises over his arms, seven spider naevi across the upper chest and moderate gynaecomastia. The abdomen is distended, and a soft, reducible umbilical hernia is noted. There is shifting dullness, and the abdomen is diffusely tender to palpation. There is peripheral oedema to the midthigh. In summary, Mr Z. is a known alcoholic with associated varices and alcoholic liver disease who presents with signs consistent with encephalopathy, worsening ascites and an acute febrile illness. I am suspicious of spontaneous bacterial peritonitis in light of this patient's history. I have started him on IV antibiotics as per hospital guidelines, sent bloods and blood cultures, started pabrinex and think that we should perform a diagnostic ascitic tap to send samples to biochemistry and microbiology.'

Chapter 15

Writing Up Your Clerking

You should always thoroughly document your findings, even those that are normal. Contrast this with presenting your findings verbally, for which only the relevant features need to be discussed. As far as the notes are concerned, if it is not written down, then it did not happen.

Best practice is to avoid abbreviations in all circumstances, although you will encounter many in a patient's notes; some are perhaps more acceptable than others.

Always begin by either putting a patient identity sticker on your clerking paper or writing out in full the name, date of birth and hospital or NHS number of the patient. If you are a medical student, it is important to make this clear at the beginning of your entry.

History	Presenting complaint, history of presenting complaint, past medical history, drug history, social history and family history should be documented as per Chapter 1.
Examination: general impression	Alert, comfortable at rest, GCS 15.
Observations	Respiratory rate; oxygen saturations (if on oxygen, what percentage or flow rate and by what method of delivery?); blood pressure; heart rate; temperature; blood glucose.
Cardiovascular	• Heart sounds: for example, 1 + 2 + 0 or 1 − 2 − 1 and 0 (Fig. 15.1). • CRT. • JVP: not raised, not seen, raised at 5 cm above the angle of Louis (the manubriosternal joint).
Respiratory (Fig. 15.2)	• Trachea central. • Equal expansion. • Resonant to percussion bilaterally. • Good air entry throughout. • Abnormal findings: wheeze, crepitations (creps), reduced air entry, increased or decreased vocal resonance.

15.1 Cardiovascular.

HS I + II + O   *Normal*

HS I + II + ESM   *Ejection systolic mumur*

HS I + II + PSM   *Pan-systolic mumur*

15.2 Respiratory.   **15.3** Abdominal.

Clear

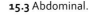

SNT
BS (N)

Soft, non-tender
Bowel sounds normal

Crepitations ℝ base

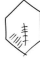

Tender right iliac fossa
Midline laparotomy scar

Wheeze bilaterally

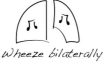

Reduced air entry ⓛ base

Palable 5 cm liver edge

Figures 15.1–15.3 Some commonly used shorthand
annotations to present your examination findings.

Abdominal (Fig. 15.3)	• Soft, non-tender. • No organomegaly or hernias. • BS normal. • Abnormal findings: abdomen distended; shifting dullness; palpable liver edge (quantify distance below costal margin in centimetres or finger breadths, state whether tender or non-tender and characterise the texture as smooth or craggy, for instance); palpable spleen; ballotable kidney; stoma; suprapubic catheter; surgical scars.
Neurological	• GCS 15. • Gait. • Cranial nerves I–XII intact.

	Impression	Draw together your findings into a summary of the case.

	Upper limbs		Lower limbs	
	Right	Left	Right	Left
Inspection	Normal, wasted, fasciculating		Normal, wasted, fasciculating	
Tone	Normal, increased, decreased		Normal, increased, decreased	
Power	MRC score out of 5		MRC score out of 5	
Reflexes	Normal, brisk, reduced, absent		Normal, brisk, reduced, absent	
Coordination	Normal, poor (specify particular deficits, e.g. past pointing); unable to assess due to poor power		Normal, poor (specify particular deficits), unable to assess due to poor power	
Sensation	Normal, glove pattern loss, peripheral nerve distribution loss, spinal nerve root distribution loss		Normal, stocking pattern loss, peripheral nerve distribution loss, spinal nerve root distribution loss	

Differential diagnosis	List your differential diagnoses, including supporting or refuting evidence for each.
Management plan	List in order of importance or priority: blood tests, blood cultures, urine dip, ECG, chest X-ray, antibiotics, IV fluids, etc.

| Management plan *(continued)* | If you are a medical student, it is an important practice to list your differential diagnosis and management plan; it is not long until you will have to commit yourself to a decision and act on it as a doctor. However, while still a medical student, make this fact clear so that other members of staff do not take any action based on what you have written. |

INDEX